ISBN-9798879187991

Cover design by: Art Painter
Library of Congress Control Number: 2018675309
Printed in the United States of America

CLAIRE ALLAN

1001 weight loss affirmations - Extreme Rapid Weight Loss Hypnosis For Woman

CHAPTER 1 – GETTING INTO A POSITIVE MINDSET

1. Every morning when I wake up, I am grateful to be alive. My health is a gift so I treat my body with the respect it deserves.
2. I am in complete control of my weight.
3. It feels good to move my body. Exercise is fun!
4. I am effortlessly achieving my weight loss goals.
5. All my feelings and emotions are predicated around my weight loss.
6. Even at the height of my pain, I experience moments of release, contentment, and joy.
7. Every cell in my body is vibrant and strong.
8. Every day I am exercising and taking care of my body.
9. Every day in every way I am getting slimmer and fitter.
10. Every day, in every way, I am becoming a better me.
11. Every physical movement that I make burns the extra fat in my body and helps me to maintain my ideal body weight.
12. Everything I eat nourishes and strengthens my body and mind.
13. Exercise comes naturally to me because staying active makes me feel good.
14. Exercising comes naturally to me.
15. God is supporting and helping my weight loss journey.

Making me feel that I am not alone in my journey.

16. Healthy nutritious food is what I crave to eat.
17. I affirm that I am successful, healthy and cheerful person whatever my present weight.
18. I always eat within my macros and gradually I am reaching my dream physique.
19. I always get so encouraged and inspired by my progress which carries me onto the next win.
20. I am a disciplined eater.
21. I am a success magnet and all my desires come true.
22. I am a walking and talking representation of someone who sticks to their weight loss journey impeccably.
23. I am achieving my weight loss goals.
24. I am active and full of energy.
25. I am awaking the giant within me through this journey of weight loss.
26. I am awaking the giant within me through this journey of weight loss. 86. I naturally see weight loss and fitness as a journey, not a destination.
27. I am beginning to see a new, leaner me in the mirror.
28. I am closer and closer to my ideal weight with each and every day.
29. I am constantly shrinking in size each day.
30. I am determined to reach my goal weight.
31. I AM DETERMINED TO REACH MY HEALTHY WEIGHT.
32. I am disciplined and I achieve my weight loss goals.
33. I am discovering muscles I didn't know I had.
34. I am enjoying my weight release journey. This time I will complete what I started.
35. I am firmly committed to staying active and healthy.
36. I am fit, healthy, and bursting with energy.
37. I am full and satisfied with the proper amount of food.
38. I am grateful for this new lifestyle change and love losing weight.
39. I am grateful to have a body capable of exercising.
40. I am healthy and lean.

41. I am learning to love my body.
42. I am loving the way my body feels as I get more and more active.
43. I am mentally and physically strong.
44. I am not afraid to say no when I need to, this will help me towards my goals.
45. I am peaceful and calm.
46. I am proud of the way I now look and my new weight.
47. I am relaxed about my weight as I am now in control.
48. I am releasing my excess weight right now. I am fighting fit and proud of it.
49. I am showing up for myself and treating myself with respect.
50. I am thankful that I have attracted the right friends who support good health practices in my life.
51. I am the One and I am the All.
52. I am the perfect weight for my height.
53. I am willing to create new thoughts about my self and my body.
54. I attract new friends with similar health goals all the time.
55. I believe in myself and my ability to succeed. I have hope and certainty about my future.
56. I bring the qualities of fulfilment, happiness and contentment into my life as I am now.
57. I choose my ideal body weight.
58. I choose to breathe in relaxation and breathe out stress.
59. I choose to eat healthily.
60. I choose to stay on track.
61. I crave food that energizes me and makes me feel good.
62. I don't have to be perfect to achieve my ideal weight, I just need to keep going.
63. I easily maintain my optimal eating habits.
64. I eat balanced meals every day.
65. I eat only what I need.
66. I enjoy eating healthy foods.

67. I enjoy my food and eat mindfully.
68. I feel good about myself.
69. I find it easy to keep fit and healthy.
70. I happily follow my diet every day.
71. I have all the mental and physical power needed for effective and long lasting weight loss.
72. I have fun expending energy through movement.
73. I have the power to change my life with each decision I make everyday.
74. I laugh in the face of challenges along my weight loss journey.
75. I love and accept myself just as I am.
76. I love and care for my beautiful body.
77. I love moving my body.
78. I love seeing my hard work pay off.
79. I love that I can wear the clothes I love now.
80. I love to exercise regularly as it gives me a positive mind and contributes to weight loss.
81. I love treating my body with the respect and love it deserves.
82. I make sure that I exercise daily
83. I marvel constantly on how far I have come on my weight loss journey and it makes me feel proud.
84. I naturally make friends who are on the same journey as me. They serve as great accountability partners for my journey.
85. I no longer eat for comfort, but for health and vitality.
86. I no longer need the extra weight to protect me.
87. I release excess weight from my body.
88. I see a new, healthier me in the mirror.
89. I set goals that are realistic to attain.
90. I take great care in nourishing my body with vitamin-rich foods.
91. I will always eat healthy foods.
92. I'm losing weight and moving closer to my ideal weight with ease now

93. I'm loving the way my body feels as I get more and more active
94. It is fun and easy for me to lose weight.
95. Learning about my body and my health is so much fun!
96. Losing weight is easy, healthy and natural for me.
97. Losing weight is natural for me.
98. I forgive myself for all past weight loss failures.
99. I Am Healthy and Lean
100. I inspire others to be healthy.
101. When I'm bored, I look for more productive things to do instead of eating.
102. All my feelings and emotions are predicated around my weight loss.
103. All the weight I lose, I lose permanently.
104. Each time I resist temptation, I strengthen my own self mastery.
105. Even in my dreams, ideas and inspiration come to me about weight loss.
106. Every day it gets easier to lose weight and improve my health
107. Everyone is different and I don't hold any expectations to my weight loss, only that it is and will keep happening.
108. Everything in my life is abundant with unlimited health
109. Healthy weight loss is easy for me.
110. I allow my intuition to guide me in the process of better health and weight loss.
111. I am a thin person.
112. I am achieving my weight loss goals. I consistently DO energy-generating and fat-burning workout routines, I consciously CHOOSE to eat healthy, and I live in a state of NOW mindfulness.
113. I am becoming fitter and stronger everyday through exercise that makes me feel great.
114. I am blessed with a beautiful, healthy body.

115.		I am changing my lifestyle to improve my health.

116.		I am creating the body I have always wanted.

117.		I am delighted to be the ideal weight for me.

118.		I am developing more healthy eating habits all the time.

119.		I am excited to be the ideal weight for me.

120.		I am extremely proud of all the hard work I have put into losing weight.

121.		I am feeling healthier and stronger with each passing day.

122.		I am gentle and forgiving with myself and others.

123.		I am getting thinner every day.

124.		I am giving myself the strong, healthy body I deserve.

125.		I am glowing.

126.		I am having faith in God and He is giving me strength in my weight loss efforts.

127.		I am in the process of developing a beautiful and attractive body.

128.		I am in the process of developing an attractive body.

129.		I am joyfully achieving my weight loss goals.

130.		I am learning and using the mental, emotional, and spiritual skills for success. I am willing to change!

131.		I AM LEARNING TO LOVE MY BODY.

132.		I am living a healthy lifestyle.

133.		I am losing inches effortlessly and easily.

134.		I am losing weight and moving closer to my ideal weight with ease now.

135.		I am loving regular exercise.

136. I am moving towards my health goals at a great pace.

137. I am my own creator.

138. I am naturally mindful of my health and habits.

139. I am proud of myself for choosing a healthier lifestyle.

140. I am quickly to losing weight.

141. I am ready to push myself to new limits.

142. I am releasing any excess weight day by day.

143. I am showing up for myself and treating myself with respect.

144. I am slim

145. I am so grateful now that I have healthy eating habits.

146. I am thankful that I am slimming down.

147. I am thankful to God for giving me my ideal physique which makes heads turn.

148. I am transforming my lifestyle to a healthy way of living.

149. I am vibrant!

150. I am wasting no energy on food cravings that simply do not exist.

151. I am worth the time it takes to eat healthy and exercise.

152. I am worthy of a body I love.

153. I believe in my ability to lose weight and keep it off

154. I can achieve anything I set my mind to.

155. I can envision my body at my goal weight.

156. I can reach my weight loss goals.

157. I choose to be slim, happy and more energetic.

158. I choose to eat healthy food in order to enjoy the positive results it provides to my weight loss

results.
159.   I choose to eat healthy foods.
160.   I choose to prioritise my health and wellbeing now.
161.   I deserve and accept perfect health now.
162.   I deserve to be healthy, slim, and beautiful.
163.   I deserve to have a healthy, happy and fit body.
164.   I don't compare myself to others. I'm on my own journey.
165.   I easily choose healthy snacks over junk food any day of the week.
166.   I easily reach my body goals.
167.   I easily say "no" to desserts, junk foods, and other unhealthy snacks.
168.   I eat fruits and vegetables every day.
169.   I eat only what my body needs.
170.   I enjoy a strong mind-body connection.
171.   I enjoy getting dressed in the morning because my clothes fit me better!
172.   I enjoy life by staying healthy and fit and maintaining an ideal weight.
173.   I feel great and look great as my body is slimming down.
174.   I feel my feelings, I don't eat them.
175.   I find time to exercise.
176.   I get outdoors and embrace the beauty of nature.
177.   I have all that it takes to lose weight and achieve my ideal body weight.
178.   I have an amazing body.
179.   I let go of relationships that are no longer for my higher good.
180.   I listen to what my body needs with love
181.   I look and feel lighter with each passing day.

182. I love and care for my body and mind.

183. I love being healthy and fit.

184. I love my body completely right, which helps me in my journey of losing weight.

185. I love the taste of healthy food.

186. I move my body every day to be strong and confident

187. I naturally see weight loss and fitness as a journey, not a destination.

188. I realize junk food is an addiction and I no longer desire it.

189. I release excess weight quickly and easily.

190. I remove unhealthy habits from my lifestyle

191. I set realistic but challenging goals for myself that inspire me to lose weight and feel great.

192. I think before I eat impulsively.

193. I trust my body and it's capabilities to heal and thrive.

194. I use deep breathing daily to help me relax and handle stress.

195. I will maintain my body with optimal health

196. I eat mindfully now

197. Losing weight makes me feel more confident and comfortable in my own skin.

198. Making small changes is becoming easier. I enjoy the feeling of well-being these changes are giving me.

199. I am becoming fitter and stronger everyday through exercise.

200. All of my hard work will pay off many times over as years go by.

CHAPTER 2 – BUILDING DETERMINATION AND MOTIVATION

201.　　　Becoming fit gives me a more positive outlook on life.

202.　　　Developing healthier eating habits becomes easier every day.

203.　　　Eating well is so much easier now that I know how to do it right!

204.　　　Every day I am exercising and taking care of my body.

205.　　　Every day I make healthy choices for myself.

206.　　　Every day I move closer to my ideal weight.

207.　　　Exercise is fun!

208.　　　I happily exercising every morning when I wake up so that I can reach the weight loss that I want to achieve.

209.　　　I accept and enjoy my sexuality. It's OK to feel sensuous.

210.　　　I accept my body for the shape I have been blessed with.

211.　　　I accept the past and know the future will be bright and very happy for me.

212.　　　I acknowledge that my thoughts are just thoughts. They are not real.

213.	I am building solid healthy habits for life

214.	I am capable of achieving my weight loss goals, and I will not let anything stay in my way until then.

215.	I am choosing progress over perfection.

216.	I am committed to losing excess pounds.

217.	I am constantly finding active things that I really like to do, which helps me lose weight.

218.	I am determined and ready to lose weight.

219.	I am developing a lifestyle of vibrant health.

220.	I am disciplined in my eating habits

221.	I am doing this, my body is losing weight right now.

222.	I am eating foods that contributes to my health and beautiful body.

223.	I am enjoying the feeling of being in control of my choices.

224.	I am excited to break a sweat and burn some calories.

225.	I am extremely grateful for the body I own and all it does for me.

226.	I am fully committed to losing the extra weight.

227.	I am going to make myself proud.

228.	I am grateful for my body and where it takes me.

229.	I am happy that my clothes are fitting me better.

230.	I am happy with my body.

231.	I am happy with my progress towards a healthy weight.

232.	I am having a healthy body which keeps me full of energy.

233.	I am in control of my thoughts.

234.	I am literally in awe of my progress and

how far I have came with my weight loss.

235.	I am losing weight now in a consistent and healthy way.

236.	I am motivated and excited to become healthier.

237.	I am moving closer to my ideal weight every day.

238.	I am my ideal weight.

239.	I am now the kind of person who can easily achieve my ideal weight and healthy living goals.

240.	I am open to loosing weight and seeing myself in a new heavenly, healthy body.

241.	I am rapidly approaching my weight loss goal.

242.	I am thankful to the universe for making me 20 pounds thinner within a short amount of time.

243.	I am very blessed to have had such an easy weight loss journey.

244.	I am willing to learn new things each day.

245.	I am working daily to achieve my weight loss goals.

246.	I bring the qualities of love into my heart.

247.	I can feel a great internal shift in my body and mind that feels so positive.

248.	I can overcome. My mind controls my body.

249.	I deserve to be at a healthy weight.

250.	I do what it takes to be healthy.

251.	I drink an abundance of water as it stokes my metabolism and mood.

252.	I dwell on all the long term positive effects that my weight loss will bring me, and it inspires me!

253.	I easily control my weight through a combination of healthy eating and exercising.

254.	I eat healthily and set a good example for my entire family.

255.	I eat healthy foods that boost my

wellbeing.

256.		I enjoy training and the benefits it brings to my life.

257.		I exercise because it makes me feel good.

258.		I feel great knowing that this process will only get easier as time goes by.

259.		I feel more alive, energetic, and healthy than ever!

260.		I feel so much confident in my skin.

261.		I find a big enough reason WHY I want to lose weight. Strong enough to pull me through the tough times.

262.		I fully commit to getting down to my ideal body weight.

263.		I give myself "me time" on a regular basis and focus on being well.

264.		I happily put efforts in my weight loss.

265.		I have a fit and tone body.

266.		I have done this before, and I will do it again.

267.		I have no fear of saying no to foods and people when I need to do so.

268.		I have the power to transform my life.

269.		I just no longer crave unhealthy foods.

270.		I know my mind is powerful, so I naturally listen and watch things that strengthen my mind.

271.		I know my mind is powerful, so I naturally listen and watch things that strengthen my mind. Helping my weight loss journey.

272.		I know my value.

273.		I love and accept my body as I release weight for my greater health and happiness.

274.		I love and cherish every part of my body now.

275.		I love eating healthy food and it helps me reach my ideal weight.

276.		I love maintaining my ideal weight.

277.		I love moving my body and getting active now.

278.		I love myself unconditionally.

279.		I love myself when I exercise my body and eat healthy food.

280.		I love nutritious foods because they make me happy and calm.

281.		I love that I feel so light now.

282.		I love what I see when I look in the mirror.

283.		I make wise food choices.

284.		I naturally attract into my life the perfect people to help my with my weight loss.

285.		I naturally love to exercise and increase my heart rate.

286.		I never miss a workout.

287.		I now clearly see myself at my ideal weight which feels amazing.

288.		I now release all guilt I hold around past unhealthy lifestyle choices.

289.		I properly chew all the food that I eat so it gets digested properly and this helps me reach my ideal weight.

290.		I take really good care of my body and mind.

291.		I trust myself fully and completely to make the right choices that create great weight loss.

292.		I visualize my weight goals and work hard to achieve them.

293.		I will give 100% in my workout.

294.		I will not wallow in the past. I move forward with joy and energy and purpose.

295.		I'm loving the way my body feels as I move closer and closer to my goal weight

296.		It doesn't matter what happened in the past, I will achieve my goals this time.

297.	It is easy for me to lose weight and improve my health.

298.	It's OK to feel sensuous.

299.	Losing weight feels great.

300.	I accept my body exactly the way it is and I constantly work on improving it.

301.	I am confident of achieving my weight loss goals.

302.	Healthy food tastes delicious.

303.	As my reasons for holding on to my excess weight melt away, so does the weight.

304.	Eating healthy comes naturally to me.

305.	Eating healthy has become second nature to me, just as breathing.

306.	Every day I get slimmer, healthier and fitter

307.	Every morning when I wake up, I am grateful to be alive.

308.	Everyday I make good eating choices.

309.	Everyday is a new beginning.

310.	Everything I eat nourishes and strengthens my body and mind.

311.	Exercising makes me feel so great about myself.

312.	Following a diet plan comes naturally to me.

313.	Food is not my enemy. I am in control of my choices.

314.	Good health is a priority for me now.

315.	I 100% accept myself for who I am.

316.	I accept my body exactly the way it is and I constantly work on improving it.

317.	I accept my body shape and acknowledge the beauty it holds.

318.	I adore the taste of healthy food.

319.	I affirm that my weight loss does not

depend on my earlier success or failures.

320.	I always get so encouraged and inspired by my progress which carries me onto the next win.

321.	I am a disciplined buyer; I only buy healthy ingredients to ensure the meals I make are wholesome.

322.	I am a naturally slim and healthy person.

323.	I am a strong presence in the world at my lower weight.

324.	I am always focused on feeling good about myself.

325.	I am attracted to the food and resources that are supportive for my body.

326.	I am beautiful, strong, and healthy NOW!!

327.	I am capable of reaching my weight loss goals.

328.	I am completely focused on losing weight.

329.	I am confident and comfortable with who I am.

330.	I am creating a body that I enjoy living in.

331.	I am dedicated to living a healthy life and prove it with my healthy choices.

332.	I am disciplined.

333.	I am effortlessly achieving my perfect weight!

334.	I am enjoying the process of being healthy and thin.

335.	I am excited for my new wardrobe.

336.	I am fit and confident in my own body.

337.	I am getting slimmer and healthier every single day.

338.	I am guided by my intuition. I know what to eat and how to live my life.

339.	I am happy with every part I do in my great effort to lose weight.

340.	I am happy with every part I do in my great

effort to lose weight.

341.   I am healthy

342.   I am intensely driven toward achieving my weight loss goal.

343.   I am kind to myself.

344.   I am losing weight.

345.   I am loving walking 3 to 4 times a week and do toning exercises at least 3 times a week

346.   I am mastering my weight loss and health more and more each day.

347.   I am moving forward each day.

348.   I am on a lifelong path of wellness. Each day I recommit to being my best self.

349.   I am patient with creating my better body.

350.   I am perfectly capable of achieving my ideal weight and every day it gets easier and easier.

351.   I am the creator of my future and driver of my mind.

352.   I am the healthiest I have ever been.

353.   I am the master of my body and my mind.

354.   I am transforming into someone who exercises regularly

355.   I am weight loss success story.

356.   I appreciate my food choices and I enjoy eating whole foods.

357.   I can and I will lose weight.

358.   I can win at weight loss.

359.   I celebrate my own power to make good choices around food.

360.   I choose healthy foods, in healthy amounts, at healthy times of day.

361.   I deserve to be slim, healthy, and happy

362.   I desire healthy foods such as lean protein and healthy fats.

363.   I do not overeat.

364.   I dress in a manner that accentuates my

features.
365.	I eat in proper portions.
366.	I eat lots of fruits and veggies which have a positive impact on my life.
367.	I enjoy every bite when I eat.
368.	I feel incredibly sexy at my natural weight.
369.	I feel my fat cells shrinking by the minute.
370.	I find new inspiration every day which helps we with my weight loss.
371.	I give myself recognition beyond food.
372.	I have committed myself to a healthier lifestyle.
373.	I have hope and certainty for my future body and weight loss goals.
374.	I inspire my family to eat well and make healthy choices.
375.	I keep my promises to myself.
376.	I like to eat light and healthy foods.
377.	I love and accept myself now.
378.	I love and embrace the weight loss journey, enjoying every single step of the way.
379.	I love being alive.
380.	I love exercising and look forward to sweating.
381.	I love living in this beautiful body.
382.	I love my body and fat just disappears.
383.	I love my body completely right, which helps me in my journey of losing weight.
384.	I love my new dress size.
385.	I love nutritious foods.
386.	I love the energy rush from morning workouts.
387.	I maintain my body with optimal health.
388.	I make awesome choices for my health and weight loss.
389.	I naturally coach myself on this journey

and am easily able to motivate myself to keep going strong.

390.	I naturally read and watching content that helps me gain knowledge and ideas for effective weight loss.

391.	I no longer crave junk foods.

392.	I only choose to consume foods that will give my body strength and nutrients.

393.	I pause and evaluate before I give into cravings.

394.	I radiate great health.

395.	I respect my body and take good care of it

396.	I take great pride in all my hard work.

397.	I will drink 8 glasses of water a day.

398.	I will let go of unhelpful patterns of behaviour around food.

399.	I will think positively and just naturally lose weight

400.	I'm free from the desire to overeat and over-drink.

CHAPTER 3 – GAINING CONFIDENCE AND LEARNING TO LOVE MY NEW BODY

401.	I'm loving feeling so healthy now

402.	I'm loving the way my body feels as I become stronger and healthier

403.	I'm now the kind of person who can easily achieve my ideal weight and healthy living goals

404.	I'm thankful for the people who help me achieve my ultimate goals of weight loss.

405.	It is so easy being healthy and eating right all of the time.

406.	It's easy to find quick ways to burn extra calories every day.

407.	Maintaining a healthy weight is important to live a long life.

408.	Maintaining my ideal weight is easy.

409.	I am reaching a healthy weight.

410.	I listen to what my body needs.

411.	Being healthy and slim is a top priority for me now

412.	By practicing a positive outlook, I lose weight more easily.

413.	Day by day, I am losing the weight and the

people around me are taking notice.

414. Every day I move closer to my ideal weight.

415. Every time I inhale, fresh energy fills my entire being and every time I exhale, all toxins and body fat leave my body.

416. I accept my body for whatever shape I am in, now. Henceforth, 'only fitness' is my mantra.

417. I ACKNOWLEDGE MY STRENGTHS AND WEAKNESSES.

418. I always envision myself at my ideal weight.

419. I always listen to what my body wants and needs

420. I am a beautiful person inside and out.

421. I am a beautiful person.

422. I am a good person.

423. I am able to release weight easily.

424. I am actively excited about eating healthy each and every day.

425. I am aligned with my higher self.

426. I am amazed at my progress and dedication.

427. I am attaining my desired weight now!

428. I am aware of healing happening in my body and mind.

429. I am becoming more physically active each day.

430. I am beginning to lose weight

431. I am committed and motivated to follow my weight loss plan.

432. I AM CONFIDENT AND COMFORTABLE WITH MYSELF.

433. I am confident of achieving my weight loss goals.

434. I am constantly developing healthier eating habits.

435.   I am enjoying exercising, it makes me feel utterly amazing.

436.   I am enjoying my slim and healthy body.

437.   I am exactly where I need to be

438.   I am falling in love with my new body.

439.   I am focused.

440.   I am free of guilt from poor dietary habits of the past.

441.   I am fully in control of my appetite.

442.   I am grateful for everything by body does.

443.   I am grateful for my body and how it knows what to do to keep me healthy.

444.   I am happily achieving my weight loss goals.

445.   I am in a state of pure wellness when I choose to take care of my mind and body

446.   I am literally watching fat melt of my body, more and more by the day.

447.   I am losing inches effortlessly and easily

448.   I am loving feeling so healthy now.

449.   I am loving feeling so healthy, slim and fit.

450.   I am loving my healthy life style.

451.   I am loving the way my body feels as I become stronger and healthier.

452.   I am loving the way my body feels as I eat healthier.

453.   I am patient in achieving my ideal shape.

454.   I am reaching my target weight with ease

455.   I am ready to lose the extra weight now.

456.   I am responsible for my health.

457.   I am returning to my ideal weight.

458.   I Am Saying No To Foods That Are Not Healthy For Me

459.   I am so happy to lose weight so easily now!

460.   I am worthy of a slim and attractive body.

461.   I believe in my ability to lose weight and

keep it off.

462. I believe in my ability to love myself for who I am.

463. I can do this, I am doing this, my body is losing weight right now.

464. I can feel my love for sugary and fatty foods melting away.

465. I can release this weight.

466. I choose to embrace thoughts of confidence in my ability to make positive changes in my life.

467. I choose to follow my diet every day.

468. I choose to make best meal choices to keep my body weight perfect.

469. I commit to loving myself throughout this entire journey.

470. I completely let go of all desires and urges to critique or judge my body or weight loss journey.

471. I crave mindfulness each day.

472. I deserve a healthy body.

473. I deserve a slim and healthy body.

474. I deserve all the good in this world.

475. I deserve to look and feel my best.

476. I eat mindfully now.

477. I enjoy finding ways to get more and more active.

478. I enjoy training.

479. I have a beautiful tone body.

480. I have a slim and healthy body and mind.

481. I have hope and certainty about the future.

482. I hydrate my body by drinking lots of water, especially after exercise

483. I let go of any guilt I have about my body.

484. I let go of relationships that are no longer any good for me.

485. I let go of unhelpful patterns of behaviour around food

486.   I look and feel fantastic.
487.   I love and appreciate my new body.
488.   I love and respect my body now.
489.   I love being slim and healthy.
490.   I love how I look when I see myself in the mirror.
491.   I make peace with the past.
492.   I naturally adopt new habits in order for me to lose weight.
493.   I now certainly see myself at my ideal weight and will keep going until I achieve this.
494.   I only dwell on the positive aspects of weight loss.
495.   I only eat foods that give my body the fuel it needs to thrive.
496.   I release all blocks to losing weight and becoming fit. I deserve to be healthy.
497.   I respect my body.
498.   I wake up each day with a clear determination to reach my ideal weight.
499.   I workout and see the results right away in my energy stamina and strength.
500.   I'm improving my health every day
501.   I'm so grateful for my slim, healthy and well body
502.   It feels amazing finding out that losing weight is this simple.
503.   It feels good to move my body. Exercise is fun!
504.   It is easy for me to stick to my healthy diet.
505.   It is safe for me to lose weight.
506.   It's easy for me to follow a healthy food plan.
507.   Keeping fit brings so much joy to my life.
508.   Losing weight is a natural side effect of eating right.

509.   I tell my body and mind what to do. Not the other way around.

510.   Consistency is my motto on my weight loss journey.

511.   I love my healthy lifestyle.

512.   Achieving my weight loss goal becomes easier every day.

513.   Being healthy and slim is easy for me now.

514.   Every day more fat melts off my body.

515.   Everyday I grow more in love with my body.

516.   Exercising feels amazing on my body.

517.   Exercising is a daily part of my life now.

518.   Food is my fuel, I give my body clean, healthy fuel.

519.   Fuelling my body with nutritious food is important to me.

520.   I accept and enjoy my sexuality.

521.   I achieve my weight loss goals because I understand the pros and cons of food.

522.   I affirm that I am working out and eating healthy to lose weight gradually.

523.   I affirm that moderation in diet is foundation for weight loss.

524.   I allow myself to make choices and decisions for my higher good.

525.   I allow myself to make choices and decisions which will have a significant impact on my life.

526.   I am a walking and talking representation of someone who sticks to their weight loss journey impeccably.

527.   I am becoming a weight loss success inspiration for many people.

528.   I am becoming more disciplined with each passing day.

529.   I am capable of figuring this out.

530.   I am committed to my healthy eating goals.

531.   I am committing myself to my weight loss program by changing my eating habits from unhealthy to healthy.

532.   I am consciously aware of my body goals at all times and I make decisions that allow me to always get closer to my goals not farther away.

533.   I am dedicated to following my weight loss plan.

534.   I am dedicated to my health.

535.   I am enjoying building really healthy habits into my life.

536.   I am enjoying my fitness routines.

537.   I am excited for the future.

538.   I am feeling euphoric about losing 20 pounds.

539.   I am flexible to change.

540.   I am giving myself the strong, healthy body I deserve.

541.   I am grateful for my body and everything it does for me.

542.   I am grateful for the body I own and all it does for me.

543.   I am having faith in God and He is giving me strength in my weight loss efforts.

544.   I am here to stay at this perfect weight.

545.   I am nourishing my body with fresh foods and water.

546.   I am perfectly full and satisfied with the perfect amount of food I need for fat loss

547.   I am physically a very active person. My constant physical activity burns up the excess fat in my body and maintains my weight.

548.   I am taking responsibility for my health.

549.   I am the healthiest I have ever been.

550. I believe in myself and acknowledge my greatness.

551. I believe in myself and my abilities.

552. I can and I will.

553. I can do this!

554. I can easily change my body.

555. I choose a healthy diet to promote a healthy heart, mind and body.

556. I choose to be slim and healthy for life.

557. I choose to eat the right foods to fuel my body

558. I choose to exercise regularly to become a better person.

559. I commit to a new lifestyle that is beneficial not only for weight loss but for higher self confidence and self esteem.

560. I deserve to be at my ideal weight.

561. I eat healthy balanced meals every day.

562. I eat only when I feel hunger.

563. I enjoy an excellent metabolism that burns fat very fast.

564. I enjoy exercising, it makes me feel very good and brings positivity to my life.

565. I enjoy exercising, it makes me feel very good.

566. I enjoy living a healthy lifestyle.

567. I enjoy moving my healthy body daily.

568. I feel at peace with myself when I commit to weight loss. And it feels damn amazing!

569. I feel good inside this body.

570. I feel inspired because I am losing weight quickly, easily and naturally.

571. I find it easy to keep fit.

572. I find it quite easy to lose weight.

573. I focus on my weight loss goals.

574. I forgive myself for all past weight loss

failures.

575.   I give thanks for having a body that is capable of exercising and effectively losing weight.

576.   I have a healthy relationship with food.

577.   I inspire people with my dedication and commitment to fitness and weight loss.

578.   I listen to what my body needs with love.

579.   I Look In The Mirror & See A Healthy And Fit Body That I Love

580.   I lose weight easily, one pound at a time.

581.   I love and appreciate my body and all it does for me.

582.   I love having such a fast metabolism that keeps my energy high all day long!

583.   I love improving my physical fitness.

584.   I love my body

585.   I love myself enough to achieve my fitness goals.

586.   I love the effects of whole foods in my body.

587.   I love the nourishment of high vibration foods.

588.   I naturally choose healthy options and lose weight.

589.   I naturally get good exercise and stay on shape.

590.   I really enjoy moving my body now.

591.   I refuse to give up on my diet goals and will persevere until the end.

592.   I regularly research recipes and learn how to make healthy meals that are made out of vegetables, whole grains, nuts, beans, fruits, seeds or other wholesome ingredients.

593.   I release the need to criticize and feel bad about my body.

594.   I space out my eating sessions and only eat during appropriate times of day.

595.   I stay focused on my ideal size.

596.   I take great pleasure in going to the gym regularly.

597.   I think positively and naturally lose weight.

598.   I trust myself fully and completely to make the right choices that create great weight loss.

599.   I turn everyday tasks into mindful moments.

600.   I use deep breathing to help me relax and handle stress so I don't turn to bad foods.

CHAPTER 4 – KEEPING THE MOTIVATION AND CONFIDENCE GOING

601. I value self control and self mastery over giving into indulgence and temporary impulses.

602. I will do whatever it takes to be healthy.

603. I will lose weight every single day if I stick to my plan.

604. I will stop snacking at night.

605. I work on my mindset to help me feel really positive.

606. I'm an athlete, capable of incredible discipline.

607. I'm losing weight now in a consistent and healthy way

608. I'm perfectly capable of achieving my ideal weight and every day it gets easier and easier

609. If I get off track, I do not beat myself up. I simply get right back on the wagon with a high level of optimism.

610. In matters of food, I am able to say no when required. I eat only what's required.

611. Losing weight is easy and I enjoy the journey

612. I feel thankful for the gift of health and fitness that is becoming such a big part of my life.

613.   I make wise food choices daily.

614.   Being active makes me feel light and free.

615.   Every cell in my body feels energetic and healthy.

616.   Every choice adds up. I choose to bless my body. I choose health and life for myself.

617.   Everywhere I look I find others excited about losing weight.

618.   Food is my friend, not my enemy.

619.   Good things are happening for me.

620.   I adore the taste of healthy food and the positivity it brings.

621.   I affirm that moderation in diet is foundation for weight loss.

622.   I allow my intuition to guide me in the process of better health and weight loss.

623.   I always attract appreciation for my slim and attractive body.

624.   I am a disciplined eater; I only eat foods that are nourishing and beneficial to my health.

625.   I am a lovable person and I deserve love.

626.   I am a lovable person. I deserve love. It is safe for me to lose weight.

627.   I am a weight loss success story.

628.   I Am Attracted To Foods & Resources Supportive For My Body

629.   I am becoming a better version of myself day by day.

630.   I am creating a life of abundance.

631.   I am determined to reach my desired healthy weight.

632.   I am developing more healthy eating habits all the time which brings many benefits.

633.   I am enjoying increased energy and self-confidence because of my commitment to proper nutrition and an active lifestyle.

634.	I am fully committed to losing the extra weight.

635.	I am getting slimmer and healthier every day.

636.	I am getting stronger everyday.

637.	I am grateful for my strong bones and good health.

638.	I am happily achieving my weight loss goals and will continue to do so.

639.	I am improving my body in a healthy way that makes me happy.

640.	I am in control of my choices and actions.

641.	I am literally watching fat melt of my body, more and more by the day.

642.	I am not afraid to say no when I need to.

643.	I am now dissolving my desire for unhealthy food. My love for healthy food is now growing.

644.	I am patient and consistent in my diet.

645.	I am proud of myself.

646.	I am reaching a healthy weight.

647.	I am so grateful for my slim, healthy and well body.

648.	I am surrounded by people who encourage and support me.

649.	I am thankful for the people who help me achieve my ultimate goals of weight loss.

650.	I am the best version of myself, and I am working hard to become even better. I will lose weight because I want to, and I have the power to do this.

651.	I am transforming into someone who exercises regularly

652.	I am transforming like a butterfly.

653.	I am very pleased with every part I do in my great effort to lose weight.

654.	I believe in myself and acknowledge how

great I am.

655.	I believe in myself and my ability to succeed.

656.	I can easily say "no thank you" when offered unhealthy food.

657.	I CAN FEEL MY LOVE FOR SUGARY AND FATTY FOODS MELTING AWAY.

658.	I can overcome. My mind controls my body. . Injury doesn't slow me down, I find a way around this obstacle to still reach my weight loss goals.

659.	I choose to be slim.

660.	I choose to eat healthy foods that fuel my body.

661.	I choose to live in a body I love.

662.	I completely understand that unhealthy foods do not help me lose weight, so I eat only healthy, nutritious foods.

663.	I consciously choose to eat healthy, and I live in a state of now mindfulness.

664.	I control how much I eat.

665.	I deserve a slim and attractive body and I am manifesting it.

666.	I deserve to be slim, healthy, and beautiful.

667.	I deserve to have a healthy, lean, and attractive body.

668.	I easily reach and maintain my ideal weight. Excess weight falls off me readily.

669.	I eat a balanced diet and I enjoy every single bite

670.	I eat at regular intervals throughout the day.

671.	I eat fruits and vegetables daily and eat mostly chicken and fish which help me gain the body I want.

672.	I engage in weight loss for the betterment

of my mind and body and for me, not anyone else.

673.   I feel good about losing weight.

674.   I feel great in my clothes.

675.   I feel satisfied at the end of the day for following my diet.

676.   I find confidence in feeling healthy, vibrant and strong.

677.   I let go of all negativity that rests in my body and mind. I choose to be positive and surround myself with positive people.

678.   I love and accept myself at my current weight, even as I march pound by pound to my goal weight!

679.   I love exercising and look forward to it.

680.   I love exercising every day.

681.   I love living a healthy lifestyle.

682.   I love the journey of health and commit to a lifestyle change, not just a diet plan. It is who I am now and forever.

683.   I love to create a fit body.

684.   I love to nourish my body with healthy foods.

685.   I make conscious decisions that help me achieve my ideal weight.

686.   I make sure that I exercise daily.

687.   I make sure to start out my day with a healthy breakfast.

688.   I meditate to get more self control to loose weight.

689.   I only think about my past accomplishments when my mind tries to sabotage me.

690.   I realize thoughts are just thoughts and they can be changed.

691.   I release any guilt I hold around food.

692.   I share with people my insights and tips for

weight loss as I know they reinforce my new beliefs.

693.   I shoot for progress instead of perfection.

694.   I will continue to love and take care of my body.

695.   I will continue to take care of myself and eat well.

696.   I will embrace my weight loss journey

697.   I'm enjoying building really healthy habits into my life

698.   I'm enjoying increased energy and self-confidence because of my commitment to proper nutrition and an active lifestyle.

699.   I'm so proud of my weight loss!

700.   I've conquered my impulsive nature, and choose food with intention and integrity.

701.   It does not matter what other people say or do. What matters the most is how I choose to react and what I choose to think about myself.

702.   It is perfectly clear to me how all the positives about weight loss outweigh the negative.

703.   It's easier to lose weight now that I have positive energy.

704.   It's easy for me to choose the healthy option that I know my body will love.

705.   It's exciting to discover my unique food and exercise system for weight loss.

706.   It's very easy for me to push away food that doesn't serve me anymore.

707.   I bless my food before eating it.

708.   I have so much potential.

709.   After a hard workout I feel incredibly proud of my accomplishment.

710.   All the people around me are in complete support of my weight loss.

711.   As my body and mind are healed, I lose weight on a regular basis.

712.   As my self-confidence rises, the number on the scale drops!

713.   Every single cell in my body is healthy and fit.

714.   Everywhere I look I find others excited about losing weight.

715.   Healing is occurring in my mind, body and soul.

716.   Healthy foods make me happy.

717.   I ACCEPT MY BODY WITH ALL ITS FLAWS AND AM HAPPY ABOUT IT.

718.   I accept myself for who I am.

719.   I achieve all my health and wellness goals with ease and enjoy every moment of the journey

720.   I affirm that I am adopting healthy methods to loose weight.

721.   I allow myself to feel good about myself.

722.   I am always eating healthy food.

723.   I am at peace with my body.

724.   I am beautiful in every way.

725.   I am becoming fitter and stronger everyday through exercise and what I eat.

726.   I am becoming more physically active each day.

727.   I am comfortable with my body.

728.   I am creating a body that I like and enjoy.

729.   I am creating a body that I love and enjoy.

730.   I am deeply in love with myself at every size.

731.   I am determined to continually make changes in my habits that will truly benefit my life.

732.   I am determined.

733.   I am eating foods that contributes to my health and wellbeing.

734.   I am filled with self-confidence, energy, and positivity when I'm eating healthy.

735. I am fit and attractive.
736. I am getting stronger and slimmer every day.
737. I am happily redefined success.
738. I am happily weighing 20 pounds less.
739. I am happy to maintain a healthy relationship with food.
740. I am healthy and happy.
741. I am in control of how much I eat.
742. I am in control of my life and that gives me more confidence.
743. I am in total control of my food choices.
744. I am listening to what my body needs from me.
745. I am losing all extra weight and feeling light in my body and mind.
746. I am losing weight every day.
747. I am losing weight for me because I love me.
748. I am mastering my weight loss and health more and more each day.
749. I am naturally slim.
750. I am nourishing my body with the food I eat.
751. I am productive during the day and sleep well at night when my health is at its best
752. I am proud of myself for losing many pounds
753. I am ready to kick butt!
754. I am slim and lean.
755. I am the master of my body and my mind – I am disciplined and I achieve my weight loss goals.
756. I can always find healthy food alternatives.
757. I choose fresh and healthy snacks.
758. I choose to be positive and surround myself with positive people.

759.	I commit to losing weight slowly and in a healthy manner. For this is the key to long term sustainable weight loss.

760.	I crave healthy and fit foods.

761.	I don't aim for perfection. I accept mistakes and learn from them.

762.	I easily choose healthy snacks over junk food.

763.	I eat balanced meals that are not in surplus of what my body needs.

764.	I eat fruits and vegetables daily and eat mostly chicken and fish.

765.	I eat lots of fruits and veggies.

766.	I eat nourishing foods only when I am hungry and lose weight easily. I love my body.

767.	I eat what I want, when I want and stop when I start to feel full.

768.	I enjoy catching a glimpse of myself in a shop window.

769.	I enjoy the taste of healthy food.

770.	I feed my body foods that nourish it and allow it to effortlessly release excess weight.

771.	I feel confident in my own skin.

772.	I feel ecstatic when I hear positive reviews about my new look.

773.	I feel thankful for the gift of health and fitness that is becoming such a big part of my life.

774.	I have a naturally healthy mind and body.

775.	I have a strong brain and strong body that is capable of losing weight.

776.	I have all the mental and physical power needed for effective and long lasting weight loss.

777.	I have an inner determination beyond food, weight, and the scale.

778.	I have hope and certainty about the future and what it will bring.

779. I have so much energy I feel like my head might explode!

780. I have transcended my impulsive nature regarding food. I now eat only healthy food in limited quantities.

781. I have what it takes to achieve my ideal weight goal.

782. I know that failure is only feedback. I learn from my weight loss failures and use them to make me more successful.

783. I let go of any guilt I have about food choices.

784. I let go of any guilt I hold around bad food choices.

785. I like to eat only nutritious food.

786. I look at weight loss as a marathon, not a sprint. Therefore I naturally make decisions that are for the long term benefit of my health.

787. I look forward to staying fit for the rest of my life!

788. I lose myself in the possibilities for myself, especially my pertaining my weight loss.

789. I love being physically fit and I lose enough weight so that I am at my ideal weight.

790. I love exercising regularly and how happy it makes me feel.

791. I love living at my perfect weight.

792. I maintain a positive mindset on my weight release journey.

793. I make a conscious effort to choose the right foods to eat.

794. I make incremental steps towards my weight loss efforts.

795. I now certainly see myself at my ideal weight.

796. I overcome all obstacles to reaching a

healthy weight.

797.   I provide my body with the healthy fruits, vegetables, and water that it naturally craves.

798.   I take good care of my body.

799.   I think weight loss therefore I am losing weight.

800.   I trust my intuition. I know what to eat to lose weight.

CHAPTER 5 – ENSURING I STAY ON TACK WITH MY WEIGHT LOSS

801.	I will always respect and take care of my body

802.	I will lose weight because I want to, and I have the power to do this.

803.	I'm enjoying my slim and healthy body

804.	It does not matter what other people say or do.

805.	It feels good knowing that all of my hard work is paying off.

806.	It feels good to move my body.

807.	Losing weight comes naturally for me.

808.	I am happy, healthy, energetic, and positive.

809.	I enjoy the way my skin and hair are improving.

810.	Age has nothing to do with it. I am releasing this weight in a wise way.

811.	Being healthy and slim gets easier for me every day

812.	Every cell in my body gets nourished by what I choose to put in my mouth.

813.　　　Every day my relationship with food becomes healthier.

814.　　　Everything is working out perfect for me

815.　　　Fitness is becoming a passion that I enjoy.

816.　　　Focusing on my physical body also helps my mental health.

817.　　　I accept my body with all its flaws and am happy about it.

818.　　　I accept the past and know the future will be bright and happy.

819.　　　I achieve my weight loss goals because I understand the pro's and con's of food and I CHOOSE to eat healthy food in order to enjoy the positive results it provides to my weight loss results.

820.　　　I affirm that I am working out and eating healthy to lose weight gradually.

821.　　　I allow my journey to be unique to me.

822.　　　I allow myself to feel good by just being me.

823.　　　I always take good care of my body.

824.　　　I am a beautiful soul with a lot to offer the world.

825.　　　I am a disciplined eater. I always eat balanced meals.

826.　　　I am a walking inspiration to everyone around me.

827.　　　I AM BECOMING A BETTER VERSION OF MYSELF DAY BY DAY.

828.　　　I am becoming fitter and stronger everyday through exercise.

829.　　　I am building solid healthy habits for life.

830.　　　I am capable of achieving my weight loss goals, and I will not let anything stay in my way until then.

831.　　　I am committing myself to my weight loss program by changing my eating habits from unhealthy to healthy.

832.	I am constantly developing healthier eating habits which brings me great pleasure.

833.	I am dedicated to being the best version of myself.

834.	I am determined and ready to lose weight.

835.	I am discovering delicious new foods that make me healthier.

836.	I am doing all the right things to keep my weight in check.

837.	I am excited and completely committed to losing weight.

838.	I am feeling focused and determined.

839.	I am filled with a sense of peace knowing that I eat healthy.

840.	I am guided by the universe which guides me easily and directly to better and more effective weight loss.

841.	I am happily exercising every morning when I wake up so that I can reach the weight loss that I have been wanting.

842.	I am improving my health every day.

843.	I am in complete control of my weight.

844.	I am in control of what I eat.

845.	I am losing weight every single day

846.	I am loved by everyone. I deserve to feel confident about my body.

847.	I am loving the way my body feels as I move closer and closer to my goal weight.

848.	I am motivated to lose weight and become healthy

849.	I am naturally raising the standard on myself and my health.

850.	I am never ashamed about my journey, I move at a pace perfect for my body.

851.	I am patient to persist with my weight loss plan.

852.		I am patient with myself and my body.

853.		I am patient with the process of creating my better body.

854.		I am powerful, unstoppable, amazing. I can achieve my desired physique.

855.		I am the creator of my own future and fitness. I determine the weight that I am.

856.		I am well.

857.		I am willing to release weight now.

858.		I appreciate my will power and my ability to manage my weight.

859.		I bless my food before eating it.

860.		I can easily reach and maintain my ideal weight.

861.		I can feel a great internal shift in my body and mind that feels so positive.

862.		I celebrate my own power to make choices around food.

863.		I choose to exercise.

864.		I choose to nourish my body with the optimum nutrition

865.		I completely and fully love and accept myself.

866.		I control how much I eat nobody else.

867.		I crave vegetables and whole foods to feel invigorated.

868.		I deserve to be slim, trim & healthy.

869.		I deserve to feel and look healthy.

870.		I drink 8 glasses of water a day.

871.		I eat foods that support my new weight.

872.		I eat only when I am hungry.

873.		I eat well, listen well, and live well.

874.		I enjoy eating slowly to experience my meals.

875.		I enjoy moving my body and feeling my heart pumping.

876. I enjoy my exercise routine.

877. I exercise to enjoy a strong, toned body. I love the feeling exercise gives me.

878. I feel good knowing that I am eating well every single day.

879. I feel proud of my hard work.

880. I forgive myself.

881. I have a flat stomach.

882. I have full capacity to create healthy habits.

883. I have the power to change my life.

884. I help myself achieve weight loss now by using affirmations.

885. I look and feel great.

886. I look forward to achieving my ideal weight. I will get there no matter what.

887. I love and nourish my body and mind.

888. I love and respect my body now and always.

889. I love setting new goals for myself that keep me inspired and motivated to keep going with my weight loss.

890. I love that I can run up a flight of stairs now with ease.

891. I love to eat healthy and exercise daily.

892. I love to exercise regularly.

893. I make choices with ease that support my weight loss journey.

894. I make sure I have healthy food options on hand.

895. I make the best choices for my well-being

896. I only eat healthy foods which benefits me immensely.

897. I prioritize working for progress and not perfection.

898. I recognize what has not been working for me in the past, and I have courage to change.

899. I respect my body by feeding it well.

900.   I take the time to really enjoy and appreciate my food.

901.   I tell my body and mind what to do. Not the other way around.

902.   I treat my body like a temple.

903.   I visualize my ideal body daily and take action to make it happen.

904.   I want to eat foods that make me look and feel good.

905.   I will be a weight loss success story.

906.   I will think positive thoughts about my body and self.

907.   I will walk 3 to 4 times a week and do toning exercises at least 3 times a week to achieve my goals.

908.   I'm loving the way my body feels as I eat healthier

909.   I'm the type of person who can eat desserts mindfully.

910.   It's easy for me to be my goal weight.

911.   It's so easy finding awesome foods full of nutrition that make me feel great!

912.   Becoming fit gives me a more positive outlook on life.

913.   I eat when I am hungry, to refuel my body.

914.   Day by day, my body is transforming into the vision I have for it.

915.   Eating right feels great!

916.   Every cell in my body is healthy and fit and so am I.

917.   Every day more fat melts off my body.

918.   Every day my body is getting thinner.

919.   I affirm that I am fasting for a day once a week to strengthen my weight loss resolve.

920.   I am a naturally thin person.

921.   I am attaining and maintaining my desired

weight.

922.	I am beautiful person.

923.	I am becoming fitter and stronger everyday through training.

924.	I am committed 100% to creating a healthy lifestyle.

925.	I am confident in my appearance.

926.	I am delighted that my clothes are beginning to fit better.

927.	I am easily reach and maintain my ideal weight.

928.	I am energetic.

929.	I am enjoying exercising, it makes me feel really good.

930.	I am getting slimmer every day.

931.	I am getting to my ideal physique.

932.	I am in control of my cravings. I eat only when I'm hungry.

933.	I am loved and supported in my weight loss.

934.	I AM MOVING CLOSER TO MY IDEAL WEIGHT EVERY DAY.

935.	I am naturally healthy and slim.

936.	I am responsible for my health.

937.	I am so beautiful.

938.	I am so thankful that there are so many tools and tips that I can use to get me fit for life.

939.	I am strong enough to withstand the bumps and bruises of life.

940.	I am strong, confident and happy with my body.

941.	I am the best version of myself, and I am working hard to become even better.

942.	I am unique and do not feel the need to compare myself to others.

943.	I breathe in relaxation and breathe out

stress.

944.	I can be present. I only do one thing at a time.

945.	I can easily handle food cravings.

946.	I can feel my body sliding into my jeans seamlessly.

947.	I can pass up junk food because I prefer different foods, now.

948.	I challenge existing beliefs.

949.	I choose progress over perfection.

950.	I clearly see myself with my ideal weight.

951.	I consistently perform energy-generating and fat-burning workout routines.

952.	I deserve love.

953.	I deserve to have a slim, healthy, attractive body.

954.	I eat at regular intervals throughout the day to avoid snacking.

955.	I eat everything mindfully and slowly and I enjoy every bite

956.	I eat foods that make me look good.

957.	I eat only when I feel hungry and not for the sake of it.

958.	I effortlessly follow my healthy food plan.

959.	I enjoy eating mindfully.

960.	I enjoy nourishing, healthy foods.

961.	I enjoy seeing myself in photos now.

962.	I enjoy the feeling of well-being that changes are giving me.

963.	I feel great.

964.	I feel the weight gently falling off of me each week.

965.	I fill my mind with messages that support me.

966.	I find it very easy to lose weight and maintain it.

967.	I forgive myself for any indiscretion I may have committed in the past regarding food. I now eat only healthy food.

968.	I have a weight loss plan and I am sticking to it.

969.	I have a weight loss plan and I intend to stick to it.

970.	I have developed healthy eating habits.

971.	I have taken control of my weight loss.

972.	I have the power to easily reach and maintain my ideal weight.

973.	I know I am able to quickly and permanently lose weight.

974.	I look amazing.

975.	I look forward to going to the gym.

976.	I love and appreciate my body and all it does for me. I now feed it foods that nourish it and allow it to effortlessly release excess weight.

977.	I love and nurture myself better each day.

978.	I love being physically fit.

979.	I love drinking water and walking.

980.	I love exercising regularly.

981.	I love how my lean body feels.

982.	I love my healthier body.

983.	I love myself.

984.	I love the way my whole life has transformed though my successful commitment to weight loss.

985.	I love to move my body and keep it active.

986.	I release temptation to eat to excess.

987.	I set a good example for my family by the way I eat.

988.	I show my body gratitude by nourishing it with healthy foods

989.	I surprise everyone with my new physique.

990.	I take joy in seeing my body transform and

my clothes fit better.

991. I trust myself to make the right choices.

992. I will be slim.

993. I will destroy my belly fat and turn my body into a vision of defined beauty.

994. I will easily reach and maintain my ideal weight

995. I will have a flat stomach and maintain it.

996. I'm amazed at how much energy I have and how vibrant I feel.

997. I'm loving feeling so healthy, slim and fit

998. Injury doesn't slow me down, I find a way around this obstacle to still reach my weight loss goals.

999. It is easy for me to lose weight.

1000. Losing weight is easy for me now.

1001. Making small, healthy changes is actually easy for me.